T0274524

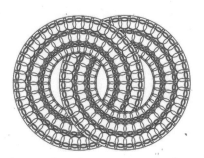

ALL THAT WE ASK OF YOU

IS TO ALWAYS BE HAPPY

ALL THAT WE ASK OF YOU IS TO ALWAYS BE HAPPY

BRIDGET BELL

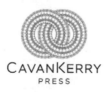

CAVANKERRY
PRESS

CavanKerry Press Ltd.
Fort Lee, New Jersey
www.cavankerrypress.org

Publisher's Cataloging-in-Publication Data
provided by Five Rainbows Cataloging Services

Names: Bell, Bridget, author. | Patterson, Riah, writer of introduction.
Title: All that we ask of you is to always be happy / Bridget Bell ; [introduction by] Riah Patterson, M.D.
Description: Fort Lee, NJ : CavanKerry Press, 2025.
Identifiers: ISBN 978-1-960327-08-6 (paperback)
Subjects: LCSH: Mental health. | Postpartum depression. | Motherhood--Poetry. | Childbirth--Poetry. | Families--Poetry. | BISAC: POETRY / Subjects & Themes / Family. | FAMILY & RELATIONSHIPS / Parenting / Motherhood. | HEALTH & FITNESS / Pregnancy & Childbirth. | POETRY / Women Authors.
Classification: LCC PS3602.E55 A45 2025 (print) | LCC PS3602.E55 (ebook) | DDC 811/.6--dc23.

Cover artwork: "Two Women on The Shore" by Edvard Munch
Cover and interior text design by Mike Corrao
First Edition 2025, Printed in the United States of America

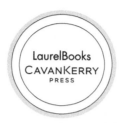

All That We Ask of You Is to Always Be Happy is the 17th title of CavanKerry's Literature of Illness imprint. LaurelBooks are fine collections of poetry and prose that explore the many poignant issues associated with confronting serious physical and/or psychological illness.

Made possible by funds from the New Jersey State Council on the Arts, a partner agency of the National Endowment for the Arts.

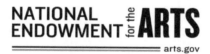

CavanKerry Press is grateful for the generous support it receives from the New Jersey State Council on the Arts, as well as the following funders:

The Academy of American Poets

Community of Literary Magazines and Presses

National Book Foundation

New Jersey Arts and Culture Renewal Fund

New Jersey Economic Development Authority

The Poetry Foundation

For Ev and Sean

CONTENTS

III.

IV.

INTRODUCTION

Like many parents, my social life often revolves around endless kids' birthday parties. It was at one of these parties that I met Bridget—we exchanged pleasantries and tried to make a connection over balloons and birthday cake while hoping our kids would be well-behaved. Somewhere in the midst of this, I told Bridget that I was a reproductive psychiatrist and she confided, or more like blurted out, that she had her own experience with postpartum depression (PPD). I hear these confessions wherever I go, and yet did not learn until much later that Bridget is a magnificent poet, who started writing about her experience with PPD just weeks after delivering her daughter.

Bridget's story is unfortunately not unusual. In fact, it's too common. Her story started with a desired, planned, and healthy pregnancy, but her pregnancy ended with non-progressing labor that required an emergency cesarean—an overwhelming and frightening experience for many mothers and families. In her poems, Bridget captures the shock of it all, including waking up with unanticipated dread, the desire to flee, immense regret, mourning, and misery. These are many of the themes I see daily with my patients suffering from postpartum depression. While no experience will be exactly alike, these poems capture the essence of perinatal mood and anxiety disorders (PMADs) better than the *Diagnostic and Statistical Manual of Mental Disorders* ever could.

When I teach, I often ask my learners how many women will give birth over their lifetime (80 percent), how many pregnancies are unplanned (50 percent), and what is the most common complication of childbirth? Most people will name some sort of obstetrical emergency—urgent cesarean, hemorrhage, lacerations, etc. My grand reveal is that in fact, postpartum depression is the most common complication, affecting 15 to 20 percent of mothers. Out of your friends having children, one in seven will experience these illnesses. There are some known risk factors, but in general, PPD is cruel and can be unsuspecting; PPD does not discriminate. In the United States it is exceedingly common for PPD to go unrecognized and untreated. During my training, two of my coresidents did a systematic search to identify articles focused on diagnostic, treatment, and remission rates for perinatal depression. They found that only 30.8 percent of women with PPD are recognized, only 15.8 percent receive any treatment, only 6.3 percent receive adequate treatment and only 3.2 percent achieve remission. In sum, more than 95 percent of these cases do not reach remission in a timely manner even with known, available treatments. To compound the issue in the US, we have rising maternal mortality rates and no guaranteed parental leave. Suicide is the most common cause of death for mothers in the first year postpartum, and women of color have even worse outcomes. This is an emergency.

There has been some progress in the last 15 years. The American College of Obstetrics and Gynecology and the American Psychiatric Association formally made recommendations to screen for PPD in 2016 and 2018, respectively. The Food and Drug Administration has approved two new drugs specifically for the treatment of PPD in 2019 and 2023. The University of North Carolina opened the first Perinatal Psychiatry Inpatient Unit in the United States in 2011, and more hospitals are investing in providing this specialized care. Still, there are very real reasons for Bridget's rage, disillusionment, and feelings of being mistreated and betrayed.

Reading this collection and writing the introduction have been a gift. These poems, in their specificity and rawness, provide texture and nuance, and help raise our awareness to the experience of many with perinatal mood and anxiety disorders. Using her talent, vulnerability, and strength, Bridget provides an education on and advocacy for the urgency of perinatal mental health—an urgency that mothers and families, current and future, deserve.

Riah Patterson, MD
Director of Perinatal Psychiatry
University of North Carolina

I.

Postpartum depression is a disabling but treatable mental disorder that represents one of the most common complications of childbearing.

—Donna E. Stewart and Simone Vigod,
The New England Journal of Medicine

Despite the recognition that the postpartum year is a vulnerable and important time, existing approaches to support postpartum mothers are lacking, especially in the United States.

—Ariana Albanese, et al.,
*International Journal of Environmental Research
and Public Health*

DIRECTIVE FOR WOMEN WHO ARE NOT YET MOTHERS BUT WILL BECOME MOTHERS

Soon you will be mired in layers
    of din, your body's smallest bones—

malleus, incus, stapes—stirrup-shaped, will shake
    to the sound of phantom milk-cries, so stop

now, while there is still this mercy
    of no one needing you, and listen

to the zip of white leather
    boots, flaunt them with a storm-stomp, like lightning

while your eardrum cracks to the bass
    of 3 a.m. dance floors because soon your world will spin

on the axis of your breasts, too-heavy cuffs, prolactin
    like flash floods, or the reverse, a drought and the body's

fuck you refusal to make milk, so pause
    in front of a full-length mirror and admire

the peach blossom, sand dune, deep taupe, cabernet
    of your nipples before new pigment paints them

a different color, admire your breasts while they are still your breasts,
    not yet udders, hold them, drape them in tulip silk,

caviar lace, smoke and ash. Soon your eyes will burn
    like cellophane, the curl and melt,

the twitch and spasm, optic nerve desperate for rest,
    so slow this down, blink, blink again, dust your upper lid in gold,

copper for the crease, smudge charcoal, sweep
the lashes jet black, cherish the body of the woman
you will never be again.

This Is How You Lose Your Body

It starts with you pissing on a stick.

The needle's prick, a glob of cold,
clear jelly smeared across your stomach.

Each week your body is named for a new piece
of fruit: grape, fig, pomegranate with a thousand seeds.

The way that you lose is kaleidoscopic: melanin
and silver, chloasma and mauve.

A geometric loss: linea nigra, vertical stripe that divides
your abdomen into domed halves.

The loss of your body is glandular, metabolic,
olfactory, it is a reverse loss, a multiplication.

The loss of your body is amplified, everything larger:
the cardiovascular swell, thick hair, and the fetus

that entrenches itself in the space
made for your organs as it claims your body
from the inside.

Origin Stories

I.
Gray smog hovers over the ridges
of our brains. We live inside scraps
of sleep, sick for hibernation's
closed-eye amnesia.

II.
The doctor complains about the cold
air conditioning, wraps a warmed blanket
around her shoulders. I vomit in a dish. Blood
and piss mix in my catheter bag.

III.
We are not mothers; we are childless
women pretending to be mothers.
We wear the mother-mask.
These babies are not our own.

IV.
There was no pain. The pain was everything.
I squatted by the garden; wetness slid down
my thigh then drugs into my veins, my slim
pelvic bone and its too-tight frame.

V.
Didn't we always want to gaze at a face
that echoes our own? But a muted haze
nets the hot, black night. Salt-rich sweat
swamps our eyes; we feed the babies half-blind.

VI.
The doctor teases me. *You're lucky!*
He laughs. Good thing it's 2014
and not 1814. *200 years ago*
and you'd be dead.

VII.
Our heads hang on our necks
like thirsty flowers, like our spines
are snapped, like we are deep in prayer
to the baby, who has become the only god.

VIII.
My homework is to make a birth plan:
lemon-infused ice chips. Massage
the perineum. Sip raspberry leaf tea.
My proposal does not unfold accordingly.

IX.
No shit, they weren't joking
when they said nothing would be the same.
Naked stomach like an empty sack
and the hyenas howling below our dangling feet.

X.
Welcome to the land of fantasy. I dream
I leave with the stars, follow their amber-iris eyes,
sneak out with a tiptoe creep
then pedal to the metal in my old CRV.

XI.
In reality, our nipples are bleeding.
Our bodies dispel
nine months' worth
of built-up blood.

XII.
Some nights I bow over the crib. Almost prostrate,
I whisper, *You have changed everything*,
and I hate you for it. Then shame
and its thorny arms.

XII.
It's like a broken leg: a callus bridges
the fracture so the bone can heal,
but it's never quite the same,
residual ache in the relentless rain.

MY DOCTOR RECOUNTS TO ME AN ANECDOTE

of a patient's vagina that *exploded,* how he mended her erupted flesh. Explains it like one might explain the process of patching a hole in jeans or supergluing a hand back on a dropped statue. I think, *When can I hold my baby?* Because I just had a baby—I mean literally—my son was just born, and this doctor is telling me a story about the worst vaginal tear he's ever seen. And because I am prone to thinking about random-ass shit at weird times, I think of my ex-boyfriend's dad, who was a gastroenterologist, how once he took me out to breakfast at a Greek diner while my boyfriend played golf, and to make conversation, I asked him about his favorite patient ever. She was a lovely woman—*classy, elegant*— who had an *unfortunate tear in her perineum, leaking fluids.* So that's two women whose bodies are stories belonging to men, and I'm worried because when the baby came out, he wasn't crying, and the doctor keeps looking from my vagina to the team of pediatric doctors that flutter around my son like he's nervous, too, but he continues on with his story: *I didn't think I'd be able to fix her.* His face is framed by my open legs. *Her husband should send me flowers,* he says as he pushes through me with a needle and thread.

Paranoia Takes Root

A rare quiet suspended between *Excuse me? Are you sleeping?*
Is the baby sleeping? Only the sigh

of the pneumatic compression device squeezing blood
through my veins, and we are alone,

no bilirubin foot pricks, no oxycodone to swallow, no warnings
about tissue clots larger than golf balls. You are milk-coma calm

so I place you on my chest, slowly, the way one places a foot on thin ice
and let myself fall asleep as you fall asleep pressed warm

against my breast. And I dream—

suffocation, alarms, entrapment,
asphyxia, sudden infant death syndrome—and I wake
in a halcyon-lull light with the knowledge
that to be near you is to endanger you.

Pressure

Breastfeeding is a culturally and psychically fraught practice.

—Jennifer Friedlander, *Subjectivity*

We cry over spilled milk,
yell *shit* at the elbow
bump that puddles the pumped
sweet gold onto the kitchen
counter. Convinced each drop
lost is an ear infection,
a diminished IQ,
we freeze the panacea
in baggies, label dates,
record ounces. When we
produce too little, we eat
fenugreek, blessed thistle,
red raspberry, brewer's
yeast. We call to other mothers:
consultants and donors,
strangers. Mid-workday,
we strip down in offices,
plug into machines, type
emails as our nipples
stretch like rubber bands. Raw,
engorged, we apply cream,
cabbage leaves, lanolin,
butter, we prop our tired
bodies on pillows, strain
to hear the soft swallow-click,
wait to feel the pull of the letdown.

RAISING MOTHERS

A bad way to raise mothers is with flyers
taped to doctor walls promising an *empowered*
peace-filled birth. Each night, a choir
of monitor lights flashes the mother's face and she cowers

convinced that she'll never understand
how to quiet the child. Sunlight halts behind
the curtains. She is lost inside the land
of it-makes-no-difference-if-it's-day-or-night.

A bad way to raise mothers is to deify
Everything Baby, to say *what a blessing,*
then hand over the flailing fists, to deny
that motherhood is hard as fuck: festering

fetid pile of bibs and burp rags,
the bottle's milk-film, registry must-haves:
wipe warmer, perpetual smile, stocked diaper bag,

love every moment, clip-on car mirror because the mother
must always watch the baby. Then it is night and I am alone.
Then it is night and then it is night again.

Checkup

Postpartum maternal health care is a neglected aspect of women's health care.

—Ching-Yu Cheng, et al.,
The Journal of Perinatal Education

Waiting, I stare up.
    Flat gray gulls painted on the ceiling tiles, watery marigold
sky and disappearing green.
                    The dirty birds scour for fragments of pretzel,
dropped pieces of popcorn buried in the sand.
                          The doctor holds
his gray face in his red hands, says *It's normal to cry. Don't worry. All's well.*

I am excavated, a cigarette butt mistaken by the gulls for something good,
      swollen-pouch eyes, C-section scar inflamed
like diseased gums.   The doctor clicks
his pen shut. *Do you think you would throw your baby out a window?*
            Sneak away to Myrtle Beach?
               No.
He's pleased.   *I'm not worried.*
              He smiles. I smile, too.
Because that is what I am supposed to do.
Two people smiling at the air in an empty room.

SESTINA IN WHICH THE WORLD FAILS TO TELL YOU ABOUT THE TEDIUM

You will sit on top of an alphabet
floormat, rearrange the foam tiles to form
words like *sexy* or *fuck*;
you will wait hours for another
adult to arrive who can understand
your joke. Who might laugh.

Afternoons of la-la-la will laugh
in your face, the alphabet
of maternal mental illness I understand:
PPD, PTSD, PPA, PPOCD, letters form
a list of acronyms, which is another
way to say that you are fucked.

You will narrate the fuck
out of everything as you walk. Cry-laugh
as your life slips into another's
life. A is for acorn. B is for bird. Alphabet
rising up from the forms
of a world you no longer understand.

The baby will never understand
that you just need it to shut the fuck
up; your husband will form
dark jokes to try to make you laugh.
SOS inked on the milk-tracking sheet, alphabet
plea lifted up to each other.

You will sing, again, another
lullaby with lyrics no one understands,
Inky binky, bob-a-linky, an alphabet

of nonsense, but what the fuck?
Why not? It makes the baby laugh:
a new joy formed.

Torture comes in many forms:
middle-of-the-night monitor lights, another
is the woman who can still laugh,
who seems to understand
exactly what it is the baby fucking
needs while I can't even recite the alphabet.

PLEA

Take this book
    and memorize its instructions
on how partners can cope
        with this
shitstorm. Keep professing:
    It will be okay.   When I ask you again,
remember I am a translucent shell,
    my shed exoskeleton   clinging
        to the slope
          of a tree trunk,
abandoned where my body crawled
    through its own skin.
Be my bones. Repeat
    the perpetual answer: *It will be okay.*
Believe me.   I am molting.   Take my hands.   I am
        a venomous snake, scared
under a rock.   Will you say
    if you think I'm crazy?   Hide
the clouds you carry flecked
    with dread. Are you scared
too? Tell me
    you're not,
        even if you are. Swear on your life.
Later, you can waver,
but promise me now that I am still your wife.

Dangerous for Mothers

after Connie Voisine's "Dangerous for Girls"

It was the summer of crumbling in the pediatrician's office
when she turned from my newborn daughter to ask me,
And how's mom doing? My hand floating

a Dixie cup of water to my lips and the doctor squeezing
my other hand, admitting she didn't love her son, *really* love her son,
until he was four months old. It was the summer of understanding

that I should be so hungry but never feeling hunger, forcing
down a milkshake and corndog from Cook Out, breathing
through each bite with dingy eyes. Knowing I needed

to eat, my mother fed me pieces of waffle drowned
in maple syrup while the baby hummed and sucked. It was the summer
I was scared to read the word *psychosis*, as if it could turn me

into the mother who strapped her baby to her chest and jumped tandem
off a high-rise balcony. That summer the OB erred
when he said I'd be okay, or rather, he said, *You have no history*

of mental illness. And I was not alone that summer—
everywhere are always women who stare down at their babies
and wish them away, begging to wake up years earlier

lonely and free. Instead of waking up, that summer I slept
even when I was awake, peering through the haze at visitors
who trilled: *We love the baby.* I watched greeting cards pile up,

pale pink and sparkly: *blessing, little angel, princess, precious.*
And then the crumbling would appear again, like a mudslide
caving in a village, and I'd drop my head on the kitchen table

and cry next to a plate of Chinese takeout. My mother said,
Maybe you need more sleep, after the OB said I would *be fine*
though I couldn't imagine *fine* while the world chanted: *Love the baby.*

Love the baby. I searched for other mothers' stories and folded up
in relief when I read about a woman who pictured her baby
floating dead in a swimming pool. *I am going to repeat what you said*

to make sure I understand what you are feeling,
the therapist explained after I choked my dread
into the phone. So, I listened, as he told me the plan

to get me better: psychiatrist, Zoloft, support group, Ativan, counseling,
sleep. I pressed a damp Kleenex into a small, compact square, nervous
        through the tips
of my fingers. And this will save me? For some women, becoming a
        mother
is not natural so much as it is gradual. And so we condemn ourselves,
        drifting
along, flashing the bright, red smile of a façade, balancing over the void
like a tightrope walker crossing for the first time without a net.

II.

Perinatal mood and anxiety disorders (PMADs) are a public health issue that has a profound negative effect on women, families, and communities. It is estimated that 15 percent to 21 percent of pregnant and postpartum women experience PMAD, which includes depression, anxiety, obsessive-compulsive disorder, posttraumatic stress disorder, and postpartum psychosis.

—*Journal for Nurse Practitioners*

Root Cause Analysis of Perinatal Mood Disorders

At the present time, we cannot say for certain what causes PPD. Most likely, it is caused by a number of factors that vary from individual to individual.

—Karen R. Kleiman, MSW, LCSW
and Valerie Davis Raskin, MD

1. Red impatiens limp in the hanging basket above a watering can.

2. Audio hallucinations, ghost-cries haunt the cochlea.

3. Reusable diapers and their sweet, ripe stink.

4. Natural birth, epidermal, visualization, midwives, doctors, hospitals, doulas, Pitocin, water birth, forceps, the abdominal muscles split apart, shifted to the side.

5. The dog's fur piling up in corners on the hardwood floor.

6. No paid maternity leave.

7. A framed wedding picture of a woman you no longer recognize.

8. The universal choir's song: *Enjoy this time. It goes by so fast.*

9. Mastitis; cracked, chafed nipples; and America's insistence on breastmilk.

10. Each stagnant week and its million days.

11. A shitty swaddle blanket that falls loose no matter how hard you try.

Postpartum Depression

a hot empty attic
  a strange fish in the ocean's midnight zone unable to ever see light
a loose button dropped unnoticed off the cuff
                    slick stones at the bottom of a river
a car-shattered deer dragging its broken body
                       a window painted shut
a cornered mouse frantic along the floorboards
         wheels on black ice—
spinning, spinning, spinning—

This is for the mother
(Perinatal Mood Disorders Inpatient Unit)

who collapses on the starched-white sheets after weeks
of no line between day and night, unanswered-yawn
of insomniac stretches, eyes hummed dry
by a screen's blue light. This is for the mother whose body is jerked
by babies that tug like puppeteers. For the mother whose husband
    doesn't *believe*
in postpartum depression, who's hit by arrows tipped with *That's crazy*
mumbo jumbo and *It's just the baby blues.* This is for the mother
who relinquishes her body to the clinic bed, who watched the nurses'
promises—*you're not crazy*—drift up like smoke
signals as they pull the laces from her shoes,
remove the drawstrings from her clothes.

SLEEP DEPRIVATION

It's okay to feel
        like a sham   like an echo   like a shroud
        like an echo
    What did you say? We said, *we promise.*
Promise what? *Huge drops, disordering of thoughts*
hallucinations. We promise *a total break with reality.*

    an especially insidious form
        of torture
    a profound assault
            so we eat a handful of almonds. There is nothing
logical in the proposed connection between combating sleep deprivation
    and almonds, but we are told to do it,
                so we do it.

We do so many things we are told to do.
    We are twitchy,
        twitchy, sleepy, sleepy, hush, hush.
    We know you're tired but don't cry.
You're not crazy. Here's a Kleenex.
We promise
    it will get better. Just relax. Just close your eyes.

Portraits of Postpartum Anxiety

I. *as Pharmacophobia*

You will not make me swallow
      that pill with its sunny-sky pallor

and its undertow voice that says *après moi, le deluge.*
      I know the bottles will flash flood me, will

strand me in a tidal pool, beautiful and salt-crusted, running
      out of air as the water dries up.

II. *as Racing Thoughts*

Each action we do
                    necessitates assurance,
because we are so damn scared we will hurt the baby.
      Please, please. Do not leave us alone.

III. *as Poison Ivy*

Once, I pissed in the woods
carelessly so poison ivy bloomed

over my thighs. In my sleep
I clawed the rash. So many problems

are worse at night. The oily resin spread,
puffed lines wound across

my abdomen. I could not
not scratch despite a lather of pink cream.

Awake, I knew each touch would make it worse,
but I could not ignore this singular existence.

IV. *as Obsessions and Compulsions*

Will I be okay? This is the last time
I will ask you. Even though I know

your answer will be yes. Even though
I know that you are lying.

V. *as Annoyance*

Half-asleep, I ignore the knock. *I will kill someone
if they wake the baby.* I am a cultivator

of silence. At night, I strip
my dogs of their collars

to mute their metallic shakes.
But now my friend's finger is tapping

on my bedroom window
and I'm pretending to be asleep

because how fucking urgent can it be
that he gets back his Pyrex, his serving spoon

from the kale salad and the broccoli fritters?
His finger is a leaky faucet

and when I open my eyes, he smiles
mouths *sorry* against the glass pane.

THIS IS FOR THE MOTHER (INTRUSIVE THOUGHTS)

who fixates on pressing the soft spot, smashed fontanelle
like a crushed gnat or a peach wet with bruised-juice,

for the mother who sees the baby slip from her loose grip,
trip down the basement stairs, concrete flip,

this is for the mother who fabricates the blue
fat face under the bathwater's skim,

who shuts her eyes by the microwave
to block the conjured thought of her baby inside,

for the mother who washes the knives quickly to get them out of her hands,
for the mother who can confide this,
for the mother who listens to the confession and doesn't flinch.

ESCAPE

Carve out naked niches, notches   in the cool stone

      day   troglodyte caves where you can hide inside

             the tile and glass walls

        encased in steam

          you are in this

     dream   you are far, far away

       floating

   down a snowmelt

      river, goose-bumped

   flesh below the water's lip, above, flushed sweat

you are pulled back   now

     to make a nest from bleached feathers, hidden inside

your piled-up pillows, you think

    of Judy Garland, her throaty voice,

      her barbiturate death   you hum

  a line about bluebirds.

THIS IS FOR THE MOTHER (POSTPARTUM PSYCHOSIS)

repeating Bible verses in the dark:
See that you do not despise
one of these little ones and for the mother

in Harnett County who pulls a white sheet
over her daughter, her son, shoots the dog,
shoots herself, who loses the mental health lottery,

splits off into the less than one percent chance
and this is for the mother who smells horses,
hears mares galloping outside her bedroom door,

who watches walls pulse like open veins,
who wears a flat affect, her face empty
like plates after dinner, who won't eat,

convinced of poisoned food, who pleads for the hands
of a deep, sparing lake. If you can hear me, I am sorry
we left you alone. I am sorry we failed you.

III.

If you ask a woman who is currently depressed how she feels about having another baby, she will likely say she will never have any more children. If you ask a woman who has recovered from postpartum depression how she feels about having another baby, she is likely to say she is afraid.

—Karen R. Kleiman, MSW, LCSW

A Survivor of Postpartum Depression Explains Why She Wants Another Baby

after Barbara Ras's "A Wife Explains Why She Likes Country"

Because eventually the gray smog dissipates and a fullness rises,
a hum laced with ache and joy. Because I always go back

for more—another helping of potatoes heaped high,
the creamy, cold nightcap—even when it hurts.

Because I learn from the hurt. Because I love
to be animalistic, pick at cradle cap, groom my infant

as gorillas do. Because I'm a masochist, because eyes stop changing
colors, because my body is already ruined, because clamped fists shake

like a colt on new legs, because the pull
of life is the strongest addiction.

Co-opting Anne Carson's "The Glass Essay" to Process My Miscarriage

. . . the world may have seemed a kind of half-finished sentence.
—Anne Carson, "The Glass Essay"

The baby's shape is a sea monkey,
a pink shrimp. It smiles and waves
little hands at me. I wake up, remembering

I miscarried yesterday. I am freshly
un-pregnant. I touch my stomach,
pinch some fat, drag

a finger across my C-section scar.
Today I am going
to see the doctor.

▽

I sit in the waiting room.
It is scattered with magazines
and pregnant women.

Polaroids of babies push-pinned
to a bulletin board. I don't want
to think so I stare at a beige wall.

The emergency room walls
were beige, too. There, last night,
I felt like I was turning into a ghost, sick

people all around me like tree stumps,
my leaking body curled up
in a chair with my thickening

impatience each time another name was called:
Mrs. Jones? Esther Jones? Mr. Alvaro?
The doctor will see you now.

▽

Legs up on the exam table, I smile
at my doctor. The room is silent,
but from the hall,

a nurse's throaty laughter. It rolls
through the walls, fills the corners.
The doctor asks questions.

My answers float up and pop:
No, it doesn't hurt much. Um, like a 3?
I search her stern face

though I already know.
A hundred baby names march
through my head. When the doctor

puts her hand inside me,
I close my eyes. *It is better for this*
to happen early, the doctor says and snaps

off a glove. I nod in agreement.
I'm embarrassed
because my blood has dripped onto the floor.

▽

I hand the receptionist a sheet
of paper. The doctor said to say
I need my blood drawn, so that's

what I say. I wonder if the receptionist knows
about the miscarriage. Out the window,
I see my car, think, it needs to be washed.

Under the window is a table of magazines:
"Birthday Parties That Wow!"
"Raise a Happy Kid"

"Ditch the Thumb"
"Nap? Snap!" I can feel
myself cracking

so I bite my lip. I don't like to cry
in public. I look up
because someone has called my name.

We're ready for you.
The phlebotomist chatters
and tourniquets my arm.

Some weather we're having,
isn't it? All this rain!
I wish people would slow down

when they drive. Clench your fist.
Release, she says. *You're good,*
I say. *That didn't even hurt.*

▽

I can't stop thinking about the emergency
room patients. Patient #1: A withered figure
hunched in a wheelchair. Stuck

into a corner. Drooling.
Patient #2: A young man marching.
Oafish. Playing the air

trumpet, spittle flying from his lips.
Patient #3: Woman scratching
and picking her skin. Her ankles

hurt so damn bad. Knock off
that racket, she growls.
Patient #4: Undetermined age.

Undetermined sex. Slumped
under a thin, white hospital
blanket, face hidden.

Patient #6: Woman watching
Shrek, her tablet cranked
so the whole room can hear.

Patient #7: Woman in a dirty shirt, too-tight
leggings, yelling *motherfucker*
into her phone. She smiles at me in the bathroom.

▽

I can predict
by my sister's tone
that she wants to talk

about the miscarriage
but I do not want to talk.
She puts her hand on my shoulder.

I know you said
you didn't want to talk about
what happened, she begins.

This is her lead into trying
to make me talk about
what happened. My sister

says *what happened* to avoid the unpleasant
word: *miscarriage*. I prefer accurate
word choice. What's the point

of euphemisms? *But, how are you*
doing? she asks. *I'm fine.* I don't know
if I am lying. I deflect and stand up.

Do you want more wine?
She does. So do I. I pour more
and we clink our glasses.

▽

The bright red fact of the miscarriage
arrives on a bench at my kitchen table.
I'm bleeding, I say to my husband.

He is washing a pan in the sink.
I'm bleeding, I say again. *I think*
it's too much. Now I'm bent

over the toilet watching blood
mix with water, and he's asking,
How much is too much? I don't know

so I go in the next room
to talk to an on-call nurse.
My daughter pushes

at the bedroom door, whining,
working hard to get to me
and my phone will not dial out,

so I try my husband's phone.
It will not dial out. I search
online, learn there is a cell phone

outage. No phone in our house
will dial out. It is hard to know

what to do
when you know are losing
a pregnancy and you have no way to call out.

▽

Hello. Hello?
The call center puts me through to a nurse.
She asks a list of useless questions:

Have you traveled out of the country?
Are you running a fever? Are the whites
of your eyes red? It dawns on me

that she may not be any help.
Should I go to the hospital?—
my voice cuts her off like scissors

snipping a thread. She pauses.
It's hard to say. I feel another gush.
Are you still bleeding? Yes, I say. *Yes.*

▽

In the ER, my husband and I huddle
at the take-in desk. I whisper,
I think I'm having a miscarriage,

and I'm given a wrist band.
We're called into a room
with a big, gray chair, a computer.

It's time to take my vitals.
My husband stands behind me,
hands on my shoulders.

How you folks doing? the nurse asks.
I'm fine, I say. I don't know why
I say this. I'm not fine. She takes my blood

pressure; it's normal.
Even a little low. It always is.
This is a point of pride

for me: low blood pressure.
She taps her keyboard
and asks if we just had sex.

It can cause bleeding. I can tell
she is nervous to ask
about sex, which I find funny

and stupid and endearing.
I make a joke to ease her discomfort.
No, my cervix isn't roughed up, I laugh.

I like to use correct anatomical terms
like *cervix* around nurses
and doctors, so they know

I know about my body,
so they might think I'm smart
and be impressed.

▽

The purple T-shirt I ordered
the day I had a positive test
is folded up in my daughter's drawer,

says: *I'm the big sister.* It was my cute plan
to announce the second baby. Instead, I give
the news like this:

*I have something to tell you
that's kinda sad.* And it is sad, but also not
that sad in the grand scheme

of sadness. I do not know
how I am supposed to feel,
so I search online to see

how other women feel. Some women describe
isolation and pain. Others prefer
angels. These options do not resonate

with me. I cannot find a space
to hold all of this so I turn
to science, read how miscarriages

can be calculated
in numbers. Hormone levels
measured until the woman

reaches the non-pregnant range.
142 to 40 to 6. In the comments section
of my medical chart the doctor writes

This has fallen appropriately,
four words that translate
to *my baby is gone.*

IV.

You are not alone. You are not to blame. With help, you will get better.

—Postpartum Support International

Pregnancy Anaphora

If pregnancy is a season, the answer is not spring
but winter: the body a cave,
a holding cell of hibernation.

Of nesting.

Of torpor.

If pregnancy plays music: the violin and its hollowed-out
wooden body, its ribs, its belly, its strings hitched taut
to tuning pegs. Its neck where pressure is applied to make a vibrating cry.

If pregnancy is a planet: ever-changing
Pluto, ill-defined, ice-rock body spinning in a dark zone
billions of miles from the sun.

If pregnancy is an animal: the star-nosed mole, a spray
of nerve endings flowering from the face; the eyes
only able to capture light and dark.

Purple, speckled bells, if pregnancy is a flower:
the foxglove, long stalk of poisonous seeds boiled down
to make the heart pump its red blood faster.

If pregnancy is a color, that color is red. Platelets tint
spit pink in the sink's curved basin. Veins like lace,
and nothing can keep that red inside the lines.

Lemons and Grapefruits

for Eileen Berton (1918–2016)

Against the silver sink faucet, she props
her head, vomits, her shoulder blades
underneath pink, silk pajamas chop
right angles into the air. Multiplying cells raid

our bodies. Fetus and tumor both euphemized
in edible metaphors: I'm a lemon. She's a grapefruit
and July is too far away. I'll eulogize
her in an Ohio winter while the paper mill pollutes

the cold, thin air. But today she is only dying,
not dead, so she can still say, *I wish I could*
meet the baby, and I catch the subjunctive,
subtle in its imagined possibility, verifying

what we both understand. July is too distant
in its sunny persistence. By then, she'll be nonexistent.

RECURRENCE WITH THIRD PREGNANCY

Following an episode of PPD, women are more likely to ex-
perience recurrent postpartum and non-postpartum de-
pressive episodes, regardless of whether this was a first or
subsequent depressive episode.

—Hannah Gordon and Claire Wilson,
Evidence-Based Mental Health

At month seven, I flip frenetic, so you encircle me
to sustain the weight of a million bees rioting

in my brain. *I'm not okay.*
You've done this before, you say as one way to make me

remember myself. I slide down
white wooden cabinets, nod my head like a flame,

flickering, nearly extinguished.
Floor tiles press through my skin, cold,

like the breath of panic infusing the room
as I sorted through newborn onesies.

The baby, a weight dragging inside me,
and woven under him like a hammock, your steady hands.

THE PEAS

Pole after pole of pea plants, thick with their distended
pods and the fear I'm going crazy again—or rather
the fear that if I stop talking, I will be suspended
in my bonfire brain, and so as to not think, I blather

to the peas. Up the poles they twist and climb,
their little, green hands clinging
to anything they can touch, through thyme,
through basil and mint. To the peas, I am singing

an off-key rendition from *Jesus Christ Superstar*, asinine,
my insistence of Mary Magdalene's promise—
everything's alright, yes, everything's fine—
the peas are incredulous like Doubting Thomas:

We'll believe it when we see it, they demur.
I shut up and concur.

On Not Waiting It Out to See If I Feel Better

When the arachnid recommences
     her sticky weave through
my brain's gray matter   I do not wait
     for the tangle

of her strong-threaded web   to take shape

because it is a goddamn lie
     to say *a spider won't bite you*
          if you just leave it alone

     to leave it   alone
is the most ruinous choice
          I could make

     so instead I heed the signal
of danger marked on her glossy body
     that hangs

upside down   smash open
     the red hourglass   turn her poison
into rubies   and fill my hands

COLLECTIVE

Remember this: inside the hard, damp tunnel of your sleep-pocked night,
there is another woman. She is across the street in the brick ranch.

She is stiff-shouldered, staring down. Inside a duplex
on the north side of I-85. Upstairs in a room painted

pink-beige whisper. Remember this: you are plentiful,
one of countless women who winces at rolled-back eyes,

white slits under thin, flicking lids. So when you incant
This baby is my baby. This baby is my baby. This baby

is not Jesus. This baby is not the devil to ward off
psychosis, the words like anchors weighing you

to this world, you are not alone.
Everywhere, there is a woman awake with you.

Apology to My Daughter While Rocking My Infant Son

it is vital
you understand my sadness   was not my fault   nor yours, especially not
yours   yet I am so, so sorry   if you carry
that cold reverb of yawning air   inside you too
the sadness   if it comes   will not
be your fault   and yet   I am still
sorry   my head tips in exhaustion's grip
watery in 3 a.m. light   as I look into the reflection
of your brother's jaundiced face   faded saffron
until it becomes your face—strange mirror illusion—
I revel in this   this beautiful hallucination
that recreates our splintered beginning.

On Beginning to Heal

To reach the raised-bed garden, I drag my body through
the caterpillar grass and fescue until I'm at the cinder blocks
packed with dirt and the marigolds I grew
to ward off pests. The flowers failed. I take a rock,

pluck squash bugs from leaves' pale
underbellies and smear their guts. Each insect
death is a heavy death, so I hush-wail
I'm sorry, I'm sorry. The necks

of thick-rind squash curve: a yellow grin
or frown, depending on the way you perceive
the contour, and the tomatoes rupture, skin
split like a wound, and the mint, sprawled green

almost to seed, spits out its minuscule purple flowers,
so tiny but tough as bullets.

Elegy with Resistance

With incredible compassion, kindness, and expertise, Bill provided care to some of our most vulnerable patients, including women with postpartum depression and those experiencing miscarriage and pregnancy loss.

—excerpt from Duke School of Medicine's
tribute to Bill Meyer, MSW (1950–2021)

The farmer's field across the road
    from your home office—*did you ever go there?*—
        is perfect in April with its shiny strawberries like red buttons

sewn along each runner's green reach. It's my favorite place
    to pick-your-own, though I surmise from the *Thank you, Jesus*
        yard signs it's run by religious zealots. Their website spotlights

a woman labeled *Farmer Mike's Wife.* Farmer Mike's picture
    is captioned *Farmer Mike.* I know you'd roll your eyes at that,
        the implied triviality of her name, that most vital bit of identity

denied, I know you would recognize it
    as bullshit, as a systemic issue, and I'd love you
        for that. I loved you. I did. I do. Death confuses

tense. Though, of course, I could never tell you that
    while you were living, cruel the way roles keep us
        from telling someone they are loved, though I suspect

you knew. I can't believe I don't know where you are
    buried or even if you are buried, death in the pandemic
        can be so private, but in spring, I will return to that field,

claim it as a place of praise. A place of resistance,
    like each time you told a new mother, *Your job is to keep*
        the baby alive. If you do that, you are good enough, that phrase

—*good enough*—a small act of subversion against the expectations
    of a world like Farmer Mike's. Maybe I'm being unfair, maybe
        Mike is quite lovely, like his field. Regardless, I will still look

the other way when my kids eat
    straight from their hands what never lands
        in the bucket, each unpaid berry, a little dig

at Farmer Mike, just in case, and I will think of you,
    how you'd appreciate that small act of subversion,
        and I will think of you each time I pull a berry

from its stem, gentle so as to not bruise
    the skin, and I will think of you, as I lug all that
        fruit home, think of how you taught me to thrive under

the weight of a new name—Mother—,
    and I will think of you as I carve out the hull and pith,
        muddle the berries into a bright, pulpy mess,

stir in cups and cups of sugar,
    a packet of pectin, to make freezer jam
        the way I hope Farmer Mike's Wife makes it,

less complicated, less time-consuming than cooked jam
    but still good enough.

I WORRY ABOUT WOMEN

in 1957 Leetonia, Ohio with nothing useful to stop
the babies from coming, from clinging to their legs
while they canned tomatoes through August heat.

And the women alive now in patches
of remote rural land, how a snapped serpentine
belt renders a hospital trip too far, how their home
becomes an island and on all sides, not water, but green
tobacco fields waiting to be cut down and burnt up.

I worry about Sylvia Plath, her sadness etched bone-deep,
eating each inch beneath the bed of her nails. I worry about her
making cookies, to cream the butter, level off the grains of sugar,
to take the time to measure the intricacies
of a recipe, and then stick her head in that same hot space
where the dough baked.

And Charlotte Perkins Gilman because I, too, ran
my hands across *the yellow wallpaper* but for me the wallpaper
and the woman trapped inside was a cockroach, dancing
its corner-wall scurry, then gone

each time I twisted my head, until one night
it was definitely fucking there. My god, the relief, to know reality
is reality. To be able to reach up with my bare palm
and crush an insect's ancient back.

DEAR NEW MOTHER—

In the future, Colorado is burning. And this time not the forests,
but home after home after home, children's charred
climbing trees so much like charcoal-sketched fingers and ash drifts
like leftover snow, gray and perpetual on the side of the road.

This I'm sure you understand: how one day you can be buoyant
inside lavender steam, your body built up to the precipice of new life,
and then you ignite, erupt, meltdown.

Everyone knows the warnings of Smokey the Bear.
The history lessons about Pompeii.
Chernobyl. Yes, I'm comparing apples to oranges to bananas,
wildfires to volcanos to power plants.

It's all the same to the people from Pripyat who walked to the bridge
and watched the flames, their upturned faces in awe
as they filled their palms with the particles
of their own death. Even if that part is myth, the end is the same.

Still, history loves romantic tragedy, which makes me wonder why
more people don't know Pelée. 29,000 died, an entire saint's city
destroyed, and the incredible story of Ludger Sylbaris,

imprisoned for a drunken brawl,
held in solitary confinement—the perfect parallel to motherhood—
in a bombproof room, safe underground while stone statues
hurled from their perches.

Call it irony. Call it coincidence, a miracle, dumb luck.
Sylbaris lived because of his prison. Call it rescued by cold, stone walls.

I know a nurse will urge you to sit by a window for vitamin D,
as if that could fix your sorrow, but, instead, heed Sylbaris's story.

Sometimes the last thing you need is a window and sunshine.
Sometimes you need to turn your back to the volcano,
search the walls with your hands until you find a narrow grate
through which you can breathe.

DON'T TELL HER CONGRATULATIONS

There is nothing like an infant to bring you to your knees.

—Bill Meyer

Because in *con* there is *with*, as in *con leche*, with milk
        and she might be sunbaked, so un-con leche that her breasts
                feel brittle
                        feel failure
                                feel conned
           as in the woman is *deceived*
                    is *duped*   is *hoodwinked*
      as in she's suspect   she suspects

the whole world has lied to her, led on
        that motherhood is *great con-grats*, with *gratitude*
#grateful   *#gracious*   so much gray   no elation
        no *–ulation*   diminutive sibling of *undulation*
which is what the walls do now   undulate   from exhaustion

        so, don't tell her congratulations
not even a *–tion* harmless, common
        suffix but too close   to *shun*, to *sham*

which is what she's terrified
        she might be: a *con*, a *fake*, a farce-momma
            so, don't tell her   *Congratulations!*

for while *con* is *with* as in *with love, with joy,*
      con is also   w*ith child*, as in the child

is now with each thought, forever, and this shift suspends
        her in disbelief, holds her in the gasp

that comes after   a toe catches   the sidewalk's uneven lip
      adrenaline-punch right before
open palms meet   the concrete's unforgiving scowl,
      and to that   only an asshole would say   *Congratulations!*

THE LANGUAGE OF BECOMING WELL

I string phonemes together to form
        an archipelago   that cuts
the surface of my impenetrable
        blue. Syllabic
landing places emerge
        from *You will be happy. You will be healthy.*   I cling
to these mantras, occupy each   word-island.

▽

Is it bitchy, I wonder,
        that Brooke Shields's memoir peels
back a layer from my sadness, that I am somehow soothed
        by the reminder   that even the most beautiful
women are not immune?

▽

Because I cannot yet create   the psalm
        of motherhood,   I whisper-sing
lyric-balms   I want to be true,
        my mouth holding the borrowed
melody: *She feeds me*
        daily soul. She talks right to my soul.

▽

Counterintuitive to crave   inanity, so rich
        the literature about social media and depression,
    but I am starved
for the mindless.   I need hashtag-hyperbole,
    meme distractions,   pretty filters
        over everything I see.

∇

From the earth-splitting   quake
       a new mountain born, and I am not alone
           but connected to
       other mother-writers; we crash our tectonic plates
       together, we form
           a jagged, brilliant range.

∇

I am nourished by the glittering simple
       promise inside this advice: remember, everything
will normalize, the verb *to normalize*—
       to bring or restore to a normal condition—
           guarantees not a return
to how I once was, but an arrival
           at whom I am yet to become.

NOTES

INTRODUCTION

Gladys M. Martinez and Kimberly Daniels, "Fertility of Men and Women Aged 15–49 in the United States: National Survey of Family Growth, 2015–2019," *National Health Statistics Report,* no. 179 (2023): 1–22.

"Nearly Half of All Pregnancies Are Unintended—A Global Crisis, Says New UNFPA Report," United Nations Population Fund, last modified April 1, 2022.

Mughal, Saba, Yusra Azhar, and Waquar Siddiqui, "Postpartum Depression," National Library of Medicine, last modified October 7, 2022.

Cox, Elizabeth Q., Nathaniel A. Sowa, Samantha E. Meltzer-Brody, and Bradley N. Gaynes, "The Perinatal Depression Treatment Cascade: Baby Steps Toward Improving Outcomes," *The Journal of Clinical Psychiatry* 77, no. 9 (2016): 1189–1200.

PAGE 1

Donna E. Stewart and Simone Vigod, "Postpartum Depression," *The New England Journal of Medicine,* vol. 375, no. 22 (2016): 2177.

Ariana M. Albanese, et al., "In their Own Words: A Qualitative Investigation of the Factors Influencing Maternal Postpartum Functioning in the United States," *International Journal of Environmental Research and Public Health* 17, no. 17 (2020): 6021.

PAGE 11

Jennifer Friedlander, "Breast-Feeding and Middle-Class Privilege: A Psychoanalytic Analysis of 'Breast Is Best,'" *Subjectivity* 8, no. 1 (2015): 75.

PAGE 13

Ching-Yu Cheng, et al., "Postpartum Maternal Health Care in the United States: A Critical Review," *The Journal of Perinatal Education* 15, no. 3 (2006): 34.

PAGE 18

Katie Nodjimbadem, "What Happens to Your Body When You Walk on a Tightrope?" *Smithsonian Magazine*, last modified October 13, 2015.

PAGE 19

"Perinatal Mood and Anxiety Disorders," *The Journal for Nurse Practitioners* 14, no. 7 (2018): 507.

PAGE 21

Karen R. Kleiman and Valerie Davis Raskin, "I Haven't Been Myself Since My Baby Was Born," *This Isn't What I Expected: Overcoming Postpartum Depression* (Hachette, 2013): 7.

PAGE 24

Dr. Kelly Bulkeley, "Why Sleep Deprivation is Torture," *Psychology Today*, last modified December 15, 2014.

PAGE 31

Karen R. Kleiman, "Prologue," *What Am I Thinking? Having a Baby After Postpartum Depression* (Xlibris, 2005), 12.

PAGE 43

"Home Page." Postpartum Support International, accessed June 2023.

PAGE 47

Hannah Gordon and Claire Wilson, "Women with a History of Postpartum Affective Disorder at Increased Risk of Recurrence in Future Pregnancies," *Evidence-Based Mental Health* 21, no. 3 (2018): e17.

ACKNOWLEDGMENTS

Thank you to the editors of the following journals for publishing and supporting my work:

> *Beloit Poetry Journal*: "The World Fails to Tell You about the Tedium" (now titled "Sestina in Which the World Fails to Tell You about the Tedium")
> *Crosswinds Poetry Journal*: "This is for the mother (Perinatal Mood Disorders Clinic)"
> *Eclectica*: "Raising Mothers"
> *Florida Review:* "This Is How You Lose Your Body"
> *Los Angeles Review Online*: "Pregnancy Anaphora"
> *Red Wheelbarrow*: "Postpartum Depression"
> *Salamander*: "Pressure"
> *SWWIM*: "On Beginning to Heal"
> *Tinderbox Poetry*: "Checkup," "Dangerous for Mothers"

Thank you to my family for their unconditional love and support: Elaine and Dan Bell; Shannon Bell and Larry Cooke (we miss you); Kathy and Phil Patterson; KB Berton and Jack Rice; Kevin Berton and Lisa Hill; Tommy Bell; and to Eileen Berton, who I wish could have made it to July to meet Sean.

Eternal gratitude to my children Evelyn and Sean for helping to usher me into motherhood. Any sadness I felt was not because of you; it was a symptom of my illness. I love you forever.

Thank you, Patrick Valle, for having the patience to tell me ad nauseum that it would be okay.

Thank you, a million times over, to Bill Meyer. I so wish you could have seen this book come to fruition.

Thank you to Dr. Jenny Detert who put me on the path to recovery by asking, "And how's mom doing?"

Thank you to Alison Schuster, Kate Pivoriunas, Andrea Ryan, and Andrea Schuster for being my safety net, and to Brittney McAndrew who gave me the vital advice that "everything will normalize."

To my badass writers' group: Joellen Craft, Lauren Moseley, Sam Huener, and Ellen Bush for helping me to lovingly craft these poems into existence.

To the coven who holds me up: Katrina Morgan, Sally Stark-Dreifus, Lauren Sartain, Erin Gallagher, Ellen Byars, and Katie DeGraff. Thank you.

Copious gratitude to my Tazewell writer's group: Wendy Brady, Pat Morris, Maureen Walters, and Button Brady (scientist as honorary English person). There is no greater magic than the magic of Writers' Weekend.

And to David Wyche, who helped many of these poems in their early versions and advocated for the "white leather boots . . . like lightning."

Thank you to my neighborhood village: Allison Simpson who was "across the street in the brick ranch" and Kelly Mehlman. I love being mothers together.

A huge thank you to Dr. Riah Patterson for writing the medical forward for this book and for her amazing dedication to maternal mental health.

To all the researchers mentioned in the epigraphs and section breaks of this book, thank you for your contributions to maternal mental health.

To the fabulous crew at CavanKerry Press. Thank you for supporting my poems and for bringing beautiful books into the world: Joan Cusack Handler, Gabriel Cleveland, Dimitri Reyes, Dana Harris-Trovato, Tamara Al-Qaisi-Coleman, Baron Wormser, Bridget Reaume, Joy Arbor, and Mike Corrao.

CavanKerry's Mission

A not-for-profit literary press serving art and community, CavanKerry is committed to expanding the reach of poetry and other fine literature to a general readership by publishing works that explore the emotional and psychological landscapes of everyday life, and to bringing that art to the underserved where they live, work, and receive services.

OTHER BOOKS IN THE LAURELBOOKS SERIES

All We Ask of You Is to Always Be Happy is typeset in
Freight Text, which was created in 2005 by Joshua Darden.
Its design is inspired by the warmth and pragmatism
of 18th-century Dutch typefaces.